ADOLESCENT IN STRESS, DEPRESSION, AND VIOLENCE

by GERTRUDE OKON BASSEY, SFCC, Ph.D/MD, MSN-ED, APN

Dorrance Publishing Co
585 Alpha Drive
Suite 103
Pittsburgh, PA 15238
Visit our website at www.dorrancebookstore.com

ISBN: 979-8-8860-4100-2
eISBN: 979-8-8860-4999-2

ADOLESCENT IN STRESS, DEPRESSION, AND VIOLENCE

ACKNOWLEDGEMENTS

Through life's expedition and my voyages of self-discovery, I gained the insight that success is never a solo feat but a gift from God as a crown for one's effort realized through the assistance of others. Therefore, for the successful completion of this book, I thank the Transcendent God in whom we live and move and have our being. I remain eternally grateful to my family whose shoulders I lean on, Justa Okon Bassey, brother and sisters. Dr. George Einstein, whose breath of knowledge, support, encouragement, and belief in me, Dr. Carla Konyk and Dr. Tulp who aided in chiseling the raw me.

I unreservedly appreciate the unique roles of the following people, Dr. Clement Inyang, Dr. Maria Helen Ekah, Dr. Florence Mandebvu, the late Dr. Emmanuel Akpan, Rev. Fr. Vincent Akadi, Anthony Utibe Bassey, Rev. Fr. Isidor Akpan, and Vero Egbe. They provided me with the needed ladder to reaching my dream.

I acknowledge with profound filial gratitude my biological family who are of great significance in shaping the reality of my being. To my ecclesiastical family, the Sisters for Christian Community, I thank both the living and the dead for making me know that the love of God has no boundary, and God has no favorite. Family is indeed a treasure.

This litany of thanks would be incomplete without the mention of "Nna mi" Very Rev. Fr. Emmanuel Efiong who assisted in every way possible. For the adolescents allowing me to share in their hidden struggles in life, for all of their genuine trust in my ability to care for them, and for giving me the opportunity to learn with them, I express my sincere gratitude to my adolescent patients, boys and girls in high school, those who had drop out from school, those who has no opportunity to enter the four walls of the class room and feel what it means to be a student. May God bless and reward all.

DEDICATION

To God. My dear father the late George Okon Bassey,
and my sister the late Assumpta Idy Eka

To all adolescents with stress, depression and violence,

My history can never be completed without you

CHAPTER ONE

INTRODUCTION

Background

In our contemporary society, teen violence is a growing epidemic. The intensity of crime rate and violence among teenagers appears to be on the increase. The mixture of adolescence, school bullying, and depression is explosive. Young people also face changing relationships with peers, new demands at school, family tensions, and safety issues in their communities. The ways in which teens cope with these stressors can have significant short-term and long-term consequences on their physical and emotional health. Difficulties in handling stress can lead to mental health problems, such as depression and anxiety disorders.

Teenage girls may become severely depressed and attempt suicide; in exceedingly rare cases, they may become violent. In susceptible teenage boys, bullying may result in depression, self-hatred, and a death wish that may one day explode in unfathomable violence. Some teens who are severely depressed and want to die may kill others before turning the guns on themselves. The context of violence in the globe is such that intertwines directly, structurally and cultural typologies of violence, with factors responsible for the act is closely knitted together in a way that defines complex conflict dynamics. While frustrations occasioned by factors relating to human insecurity and obnoxious policies, among others, largely define structural violence, the physical expression of such development is in a form of verbal and physical attacks resulting in physical harms and killings largely describe direct violence. At times, the perpetrators of such direct violence attempt to justify their actions on deconstructed religious sentiments, customs, traditions, and cultural beliefs, while others anchor their justifications on conditions of human insecurity such as joblessness, hunger, and environmental problems among others. The pattern and complexity of the violence in some parts of the world is in fact worrisome as the nation-state seems to be teetering at the verge of precipice. It is against this backdrop that this book aims at examining the nature and extent of violence among stressed and depressed teenagers. The baffling episodes involving adolescents-turned-killers raise disturbing questions: What leads school-age children to committing unconscionable acts of violence against their peers? As parents, we ponder the troubling question of what could possibly inspire a teenage—middle-class—to plot and indeed, carry out a minutely detailed plan to assassinate or massacre his fellow students.

Consequently, the etiologic significance of exposure to any single type of violence is unclear. An alternative approach to this problem is to consider the patterns of violence that adolescents are mostly exposed to and then to determine which patterns are most deleterious for child and adolescent mental health.

Teen violence experiences

Violence is any physical conduct that causes injury or harm to another person. Teen violence means that either the victim, the perpetrator, or both are between twelve and twenty years old. Teen violence includes murder, shooting, stabbing, beating, rape, robbery, and even simply threatening someone with physical harm. All are against the law.

The terms *teen*, *youth*, and *juvenile* are used interchangeably when discussing violence by and against young people. A teen is a person between thirteen and twenty years old. Youth is a more general term applied to individuals between ages twelve and twenty-four. Juvenile has a precise meaning, especially to police and judges, since the Federal Bureau of Investigation (FBI) officially defines juvenile crime as illegal acts committed by persons ages ten through seventeen.

Risk for Witnessing Violence and Violence Victimization

Stories of violence by and against youth explode from the news like gunshots from a passing car. America is under attack by armed teenagers.[1] Historically, national surveillance data indicate that witnessing violence and violence victimization are common for youth in the United States,[2] and these experiences can occur within any setting where youth spend time (e.g., home, school, and neighborhood). For example, an estimated 3–10 million children witness intimate partner violence each year[3], and 28.4% of adolescents in the National Longitudinal Study of Adolescent Health reported physical assault by caregivers during childhood. In 2007, 5.4% of female high school students and 10.2% of male high school students reported that they were threatened or injured with a weapon on school property at least once in the past years; and 5.5% of high school students nationwide had not attended school at least one time in the previous 30 days because they felt that they would be unsafe on their way to school or while in school.[4]

Comparably, the Nigerian situation is not very different. The Nigerian history is dotted with stories of violence. Going by the annals of records, different natures of violence ranging from ethno-religious conflicts to indigenes-settlers' conflicts, Niger Delta resource-based conflict to Boko Haram violence menace, and communal mayhem over land dispute to farmers/cattle- rearers' conflicts, as well as gender, school-based violence and electoral cum political violence among others, have at various extent affected the progress and peaceful co-existence of the good people of Nigeria. Worst of all the violence in recent time is the Boko Haram suicide bombing campaign in the northeastern part of the country. Importantly, the risk for witnessing violence and violence victimization varies across the adolescent population, and not all adolescents face the same risk for exposure.

Studies show that youth exposure to violence is associated with several individual, family, and community characteristics, including age, gender, race, family socioeconomic status (SES), parental mental health and substance use, and neighborhood characteristics. Considering community violence, witnessing or violence victimization is more common among boys, youth from poorer families, and racial/ethnic minority youth, and exposure tends to increase with age.[5]

Moreover, individuals often experience co-occurring forms of violence within a given period of time. For instance, children who witness intimate partner violence could also experience child maltreatment, and family violence is more frequently reported in disadvantaged neighborhoods.[6]

Violence and Mental Health of Teens.

To develop interventions and policies that protect children and adolescents, it is important to have comprehensive information about youth violence experiences, including knowledge about the most common and harmful patterns of exposure. There are several strategies that researchers have used to evaluate the association between multiple co-occurring forms of violence and mental health outcomes. Perhaps the most common approach is to include multiple measures of violence experiences in a single regression model and to estimate the "independent" associations of each type of violence with subsequent mental health.[7]

However, a drawback of this approach is that the independent associations between each type of violence and mental health (controlling for all other types of violence) are not informative about the impact of multiple exposures on mental health. In theory, one could use the results from these models to estimate the predicted probabilities of disorders (or mean levels of symptoms) associated with hypothetical combination of exposure. However, these results still would not tell us which combinations of exposures are most prevalent and what the risk of disorders associated with each combination is.

CHAPTER TWO

EXPOSURE TO VIOLENCE
AND DEPRESSIVE OUTCOMES IN TEENS

Exposure to violence is associated with several negative outcomes. Youth exposed to violence are more likely to have economic disadvantage, criminal victimization, and criminal perpetration.[8] In one study, 29% of youth from a Southern metropolitan community who were exposed to violence reported clinical levels of post-traumatic stress disorder (PTSD).[9] Furthermore, in a meta-analysis of 41 studies examining the effects of exposure to violence, researchers found that those exposed to violence were at an increased risk for both internalizing and externalizing behaviors.[10] Although we know of some of the repercussions of exposure to violence, much remains to be learned.

Violence is a complex phenomenon involving individuals, interpersonal relationships, communities, and society.[11] Violence has become a major public health issue over the past decades, since it has been found to be a worthy cause of mortality and morbidity worldwide. According to the World Health Organization (WHO),[12] more than 1.6 million people died in 2000 because of violence. More than 90% of these deaths occurred in low and middle-income countries (LAMIC). Violence rates are particularly high in the Americas, where the average rates of homicide for the years 2000-2004, estimated at 17.8 homicides per 100,000 inhabitants,[13] was the highest in the world.

There exist numerous challenges associated with understanding the influences of stress and depression on young people who turn out to be violent. Depression often lurks just beneath the surface of even the most violent act. *"If you do a role play with batterers and freeze the action before the lashing out and ask them how they feel, they'll say they feel betrayed, unloved. There's a millisecond of tolerance for those depressive feelings, and then the man flips up into dominance rage and lashes out,"* says Terrence Real, a Cambridge-based psychotherapist who works with perpetrators of abuse. It might seem that such rage disappears with the onset of depression, but studies show that's not the case. According to a recent report in the Journal of Clinical Psychiatry, about one in three depressed people are also openly hostile. In addition, many depressed people have "anger attacks"—characterized by a racing heartbeat, sweating, hot flashes, and a tightness in the chest—in response to even minor irritations. More than 60 percent of depressed patients who have anger attacks say they have physically or verbally attacked others during their fits of rage, according to the report. The deterioration of security situation and violence in certain parts of the world especially in Nigeria has increased in recent times. While the rights of children remain unprotected by the government, forced evictions are spreading to the nooks and crannies of the country. According to Human Right Watch (2011), more than 14,500 people have lost their lives due to inter-communal, political, and sectarian violence since 1999 when the military regimes gave way to democratic Government in Nigeria. As a result of widespread poverty and poor governance, militant groups have continued to thrive resulting in killings and reign of violence. Little is known about any possible roots and causes of violence in individuals especially teens, or in society.

With all the apparent wide-ranging effects of violence, some caution should be exercised, looking into the root causes.

UNDERSTANDING THE ASSOCIATION OF VIOLENCE EXPOSURE

Domains of violence

Teen violence is common where young people live, particularly in the nation's troubled urban areas. Some geographical areas of the country have a higher incidence of teen violence than others. The only thing that these regions have in common is that they all include large urban areas. In many cities, some neighborhoods seem like war zones, and the teens who live there are both the soldiers and the victims. Still, some cities have much higher rates of juvenile violence than others.

The 1995 FBI report on national arrest figures showed five urban areas with juvenile violent crime arrest rates over 1,000 per 100,000 juveniles: Hudson County (Jersey City), New Jersey (1,302); New York City, New York (1,247); San Francisco, California (1,080); Racine, Wisconsin (1,059); and Fulton County (Atlanta), Georgia (1,056). Although these areas have prominent juvenile crime rates that exceed 1 percent of their juvenile populations, violent crime is increasing in all parts of the country. Between 1984 and 1994, the average of violent crime arrests per 100,000 juveniles in all rural areas went from 46 to 135, in all suburban areas from 102 to 236, and in all urban areas from 150 to 540.[14]

Violence at School

City school grounds are a frequent site of teen violence. As an indicator of how big the problem is, the security personnel for New York City schools make up the ninth-largest police force in the nation, reported Martin Haberman and Vicky Dill in the Summer 1995 issue of *Educational Forum*. In a 1995 study reported in *USA Today*, Arlene Stiffman, a professor at the George Warren Brown School of Social Work, found one-third of inner-city students said they had seen at least one physical attack or robbery involving teens on campus during the preceding year, and 25 percent said that teachers at their school had been injured by students.

Furthermore, the study indicated that the neighborhoods near inner-city schools tended to be more dangerous than other nearby similar areas that were not near schools.

A 1995 report by the American Federation of Teachers found that during the previous year more than 3 million students nationwide reported being assaulted or threatened with assault at school, and that the daily average number of children who did not attend school because they were afraid of being attacked was approximately 160,000. Teachers across the country also reported that they were forced to spend much of their time in class defusing potentially violent problems, which left less time for teaching and learning.[15]

Violence at home (Domestic Violence)

Another place where teen violence is especially likely to occur is inside the home. Statistics confirm that violence—spouse abuse, child abuse, beatings—inside the home is widespread. Different terms have been used to describe children who have been exposed to domestic violence. Early research often described children as being "witnesses" or "observers" of such violence; more recently, however, researchers have begun to use the term "exposure" to domestic violence.[16] Within the empirical literature, however, few studies articulate what is meant by "childhood exposure" and many do not report information about the type or extent of violence to which the child is exposed. Thus, to date, no standardized definition of childhood exposure to violence has emerged.[17] Despite such lack of consensus, most researchers agree that exposure to domestic violence occurs when children see, hear, are directly involved in (i.e., attempt to intervene), or experience the aftermath of physical or sexual assaults that occur between their caregivers.[18]

A 1996 study by the National Centre on Child Abuse and Neglect (a department of the U.S. Department of Health and Human Services) revealed that in over half of the families in which the adult woman is physically abused by the adult man, the children are also physically assaulted. The study also concluded that children from violent homes are almost twice as likely to engage in violence as children from homes where there is no physical abuse.

In 1995 over 3 million children were reported abused or neglected in the United States, according to a state-by-state survey conducted by the National Committee to Prevent Child Abuse. That represented a rise of 2 percent over the 1994 figure. Furthermore, a 1996 report by the U.S. Department of Health and Human Services found that the number of child abuse and neglect cases nearly doubled between 1986 and 1993 to 2.8 million cases, and that is just the cases that were reported. A 1995 Gallup poll of parents found that physical abuse may be as much as six times higher than the official reported number and sexual abuse may be ten times higher. Events within a family that leave a person injured physically or mentally or that result in death are not just a "family matter" in the eyes of the courts. Family violence is a crime.[19]

Developmental factors moderating the effects of exposure to domestic violence

Gender as a moderator of the outcomes of exposure to domestic violence

Gender-based violence is an age-old psycho-social issue deeply rooted in the dwindling concept of gender inequality which is a kind of structural violence within any social system. Gender-based violence is broadly used as "violence against women and it also highlights gender inequality in which most violence is rooted" (USAID, 2006, p.66). The Beijing Declaration and the Platform for Action defined it as "any act of gender-based violence that results in, or is likely to, result in physical, sexual, or psychological harm or suffering to women including threats of such acts, coercion or arbitrary deprivation of liberty whether occurring in public or private life. Among the various forms of violence against women are battering by spouse, rape, verbal assault, female genital mutilation, incest, child marriage, forced marriage, denial of women work opportunity, denial of women's right to own property, denial of girl child right to choose her husband, denial of girl child access to education, child labor, girl child trafficking and using girl child for commercial sex purposes, among others.

CHAPTER FOUR

Forms of Violence

Murder

In 1989, the FBI reported that 11 percent of all murders (homicides) in the United States were committed by kids under the age of eighteen. In 1992 that figure had climbed to almost 15 percent. Two years later it was 17 percent. Nationally, the number of juveniles who killed another person with a handgun quintupled between 1984 and 1994 (358 to 1,856, more than a 500 percent increase), according to a North-Astern University report submitted to the U.S. Attorney General. And the Centre to Prevent Handgun Violence reported that in 1995, 78 percent of all killings in which the victims were between thirteen and twenty were committed with guns.

Assault and Robbery

The figures for juvenile violent crimes other than murder have also been climbing. From 1985 to 1994, the number of all violent crimes handled by juvenile courts doubled to fifty-four hundred cases. Compared with 1985, in 1994 juvenile courts handled 25 percent more rape cases, 53 percent more robbery cases, 134 percent more aggravated assault cases, and 91 percent more simple assault cases. During the same period, juvenile courts saw violations of gun laws increase 156 percent.

A simple assault is an attack, or a threatened attack, directed toward another person without using a deadly weapon. An aggravated assault is an attack, or a threatened attack directed toward another person with the intention of hurting or killing that person with a deadly weapon. Robbery is an assault, simple or aggravated, with the intention of depriving another person of property or money. Unlike other categories of violent crime, serious assaults by juveniles remained at a constant rate from 1965 to the mid-1990s (between 9 and 12 percent of all reported cases). Juveniles were charged with committing 16 percent of all reported robberies in 1992.

Rape and Dating Violence

According to crime experts, most adult rapists begin their sexual violence during adolescence or even younger. FBI figures show that boys younger than eighteen account for 14 percent of all rape arrests in the United States. That translates to four thousand and in some instances five thousand juvenile arrests for rape each year. Over 5 percent of those boys are age fifteen and under. Rape is often the ultimate result of what is known as dating violence. Dating violence ranges from verbal abuse to a slap in the face to harsher physical abuse including rape and even murder committed in a fit of jealous rage. The chief characteristic of dating violence is that there is sex and/or physical harm that is unwanted by one of the individuals.

The overwhelming majority of perpetrators of dating violence are male, which explains why dating violence is sometimes called boyfriend violence. According to a 1996 report from the Family Research Laboratory at the University of New Hampshire, up to 28 percent of teenagers in an intimate relationship are affected by dating violence. In another study conducted in 1992 at the University of Illinois, 36 percent of high school girls reported they had experienced violence on a date. Dating violence is reported with nearly equal frequency in cities, towns, and suburban areas, according to the U.S. Department of Justice, and it cuts across all racial and ethnic lines. But teens from families with incomes in the poverty range report the most cases, with the numbers decreasing with higher education and income levels. In nearly all situations, however, dating violence is an aspect of teenage life that is usually hidden from parents or other adults.

Of the high school girls who reported dating violence to the researchers in the Illinois study, only 4 percent had talked about it with a parent or other authority figure. A few had told peers, but almost all had remained silent.

Consequences of Violence

Violence perpetration

Researchers often state that exposure to violence is a risk factor for later violent perpetration and victimization, but this assertion has not been tested adequately. **The 2001 Surgeon General's Report states**: *"Studies have shown that adolescents exposed to violence are more likely to engage in violent acts,"* and then goes on to cite several studies, none of which tested this relationship (pg. 1902). Cited in the report, Fagan & Wilkinson (1998) discuss how exposure to violence should, theoretically, lead to violence given a script framework, but they did not actually conduct such a study (Fagan & Wilkinson, 1998). Another cited study in the report linked exposure to violence to symptoms of psychological trauma, but not to violent behaviors (Singer, Anglin, Song, & Lunghofer, 1995). Other researchers that are frequently cited when linking exposure to violence with subsequent violent behaviors have yielded inconsistent results (Finkelhor et al., 2005) with several researchers reporting no significant relationships (Feigelman, Howard, Li, & Cross, 2000). These inconsistencies may result from studies of varying timeframes and measurement. To best understand the association between exposure to violence and violence perpetration, a cross-developmental study is needed that accounts for concurrent exposures to violence.

While prior researchers have found inconsistencies when studying the association between violence exposure and violent behaviors, such an association can be explained by social cognitive theory and scripts theory. According to Bandura's social cognitive theory, behaviors and attitudes are learned through observation.[20] In conjunction with social cognitive theory, script theory posits that youth learn scripts through observation, which are then activated when environmental cues arise.[21] Taken together, these two theories provide support for the notion that exposure to violence may engender the use of violence. I hypothesize that those with high or medium exposure to violence profiles in late adolescence are more likely to use violence to solve problems later in life.

Depression:
To a young person, being exposed to violence can be interpreted to mean that their community and world are unsafe, and that they are unworthy of being protected.[22] Among the host of negative repercussions associated with exposure to violence, internalizing symptoms are often cited.[23] Internalizing problems refer to somatic complaints, problems of withdrawal, and anxiety or depression.[24] Youth exposed to violence are less likely to talk with others about stress-related concerns and thoughts, thereby increasing their risk for anxiety and depression. If left untreated, depression can increase one's risk of suicide, addiction, self-injury, reckless behavior, relationship problems, and health concerns.[25] Yet, when researchers have specifically investigated the relationship between exposure to violence and depression, they have yielded inconsistent findings.[26] For example, Gorman-Smith & Tolan found that among 245 Latino and African American boys from a disadvantaged community in Chicago, exposure to violence increased depression over a one year period.[27] In a different cross-sectional sample of 185 high school students from poor inner-city school, youth exposed to chronic community violence were more likely to display internalizing behaviors (i.e., somatic complains, withdrawn behavior), but not depressive symptoms.[28] Finally, in a cross-sectional study of 251 youth from an economically-disadvantaged community, researchers found that the relationship between exposure to violence and depression was curvilinear.[29]

America vis-à-vis Nigeria

Figures from the World Health Organization's National Centre for Health Statistics show the level of youth violence varies greatly from country to country. The WHO's 1994 homicide rates (murders per 100,000 people) for males aged fifteen to twenty-four, listed highest to lowest, were: United States, 21.9; Scotland, 5.0; New Zealand, 4.0; Israel, 3.7; Canada, 2.9; France, 1.4; Greece, 1.4; Ireland, 1.2; Poland, 1.2; Great Britain, 1.2; Japan, 0.5. Clearly the United States leads the industrialized world in violent youth crime, but it is also in a league by itself in the number of deaths caused by shooting. According to the Centre to Prevent Handgun Violence, in 1990 the number of deaths caused by handguns (including homicides and accidents) in some representative countries were: United States, 10,567; Switzerland, 91; Japan, 87; Great Britain, 22; Australia, 10. Furthermore, according to the United Nations Interregional Crime and Justice Research Institute, the United States has the highest statistics in other areas that affect teen violence, including child poverty, crime, and imprisonment. Compared with Europe, for example, the United States has more than twice as much child poverty and crime per 100,000 people, and more than five times as many of its citizens are imprisoned.

The story is not very different in Nigeria. Since her independence in 1960, there is hardly any region in Nigeria that has not experienced one form of violence or the other. The diversity some believe is one of the sources of the country's strength while several other people believe it is the gunpowder to many violent conflicts in the country. By and large, the country which is the largest community of blacks in the world has despite the plethora of challenges continued to forge ahead in unity as a nation-state. Apart from the civil war, the Niger Delta violence, Fulani Herdsmen, cultism, and the Boko Haram violence are the most prominent and protracted violent conflicts that have brought the economy of the country to her kneel.

The importation of suicide bombing by the Boko Haram sect changed the dynamics and the pattern of violence unleashing in the country. Though the Boko Haram activities have been largely localized in the northeastern part of the country, the entire country is however suffering from the consequences of the violence that is fast soiling the good image of the country among international communities. Also, there have been pockets of human rights violation and unlawful killings including torture and enforced disappearance and ill-treatment (Amnesty International Report, p.2011) in some parts of the country especially in the northeast.

Over the years, ethno-religious conflict also largely dotted the Nigerian communities. The employment of religion as an instrument for fomenting violence in Nigeria's polity is traceable to the era of the British colonialists whose colonial administrations intentionally exploited religion as an instrument of pacification in the country. Violence in Jos has continued through the era of the military junta into the democratic regimes which has also been overwhelmed by political muscle, centrifugal divisions and ethno-religious polarizations including weak governance. It is believed by some scholars that the multi-ethnic, multi-religious, multi-linguistic and multi-cultural nature of the Nigerian society may also be serving as catalyst for the frequent occurrence of violence. There are over 250 ethnic groups with their unique cultures, and as posited by IDEA (2001, p.87) *"ethnic culture is one of the important ways people conceive of themselves, and culture and identity are closely intertwined"*. In Nigeria, ethnic cultures have been wrongly exploited to brand the country with tribalism, and manipulation of religious sentiments as well as regionalism largely explains the unequal development of the country, and this, in addition to the perennial social tension and political instability because of ethnic sectarianism, has left a trail of destructive violence and even *"threatened the territorial integrity of Nigeria"* (IDEA, 2001, p.89).

Gender-based violence is another common type of violence in Nigeria. Gender describes behaviors, attributes or characteristics and roles expected in the society of individuals based on being born of male or female (Uwameiye and Iserameiya, 2013, p.219) and gender-based violence is most often against the women and the girl child, and mainly within the family. Gender-based violence manifests in different forms such as physical, sexual, economic, emotional, mental, and psychological. However, the physical aspect is the most prevalent of the various forms of intimate partner violence. Intimate partner violence is often cloaked with denial, shame, and silence by the victims, and it occurs between two persons in a close relationship whether current spouse or erstwhile spouse or dating partners. It is the *"actual or threatened physical or sexual violence or psychological and emotional abuse directed toward a spouse, ex- spouse, current or former boyfriend or girlfriend, or current or former dating partner"* (Saltzman et al. 2002, p.10), and it is increasingly replacing the term domestic violence (WHO, 2005a).

CHAPTER FIVE

Drug Abuse; Major Cause of Violence Among Teens in Nigeria

The National Drug Law Enforcement Agency (NDLEA) said recent statistics have revealed that 40 percent of Nigerian youth are deeply involved in the abuse of drugs. The prevalence of drug abuse in Nigeria and the negative impact on public health and safety necessitate that all hands must be on deck to curtail the challenge in our country. There is no better time than now for all relevant stakeholders to rise to the fight and join the crusade the NDLEA is leading to make our country a better place and safer nation especially for the youths who are the leaders of tomorrow.

The prevailing culture of drug abuse has in no small measure contributed to the upsurge in youths' violence. Hard drugs such as heroin, marijuana and cocaine are often found in the possession of youths. Violence clashes often occur under the influence of these drugs and alcohol. *Ifatuorti [1994:156]* attest to the fact that abuse drugs such as cocaine and over- indulgence in alcoholic drink such as gin, whisky and beer alter state of the user's mind and predispose them to violence

On the study of drug use among young people in Nigeria, the study included a sample of 2,846 students from 17 secondary schools in Lagos, the other 300 patients admitted to Lagos University teaching hospital for treatment of drug abuse. Among the secondary school students, the major substances used were alcohol, barbiturates central and cannabis and also the major patients treated were cannabis users.

With this kind of situation and alarming rate in which teens abuse drugs, what therefore can remedy the situation?

In an attempt to conceptualize youth violence and the context within which the problem is produced in Nigeria, *Hon. Agu F.C. of the department of political science, Caritas University, Enugu State*, in his work analyzes youth involvement in violence as manifested in Nigeria is evidence of the teens not a having a proper upbringing, unemployment, poverty, government not implementing policies to help parenting and child abuse among other causative factors. Such violence often poses serious challenges to human development in the 21st century Nigeria. Hence, the need for an urgent measure to address the menace. Towards addressing the problems of youth violence in Nigeria, therefore the following suggestions are hereby proffered. The government at all levels must dissociate themselves from violence and from those who maintain their positions through coercion. There is no doubt that government supportive of violence will only continue to promote violence rather than reducing the menace.

Since the youths are the leaders of tomorrow, special efforts should be made to encourage and promote activities that are of interest to the young minds in a way to promote tolerance, trust and cosmopolitanism among them. These call for the strengthening of cross religious and ethnic institutions for youth developmental programs like sporting activities across the primary and secondary schools, this kind of engagement will help to develop their mindset positively to encourage healthy competition among them. It is certain that if the young minds are not positively groomed, the nation is heading of destruction and stagnation.

Teens should be encouraged to develop a culture of reading books that can challenge them to be better leaders and good ambassadors for the society at large representing and portraying a good image for us all, this in turn brings development and stability to the nation.

CHAPTER SIX

Media Exposure and Internet Content; Influencer to Teens Behaviour

Research indicates that violence in the media influences teens and causes them to act aggressively. Although it is difficult to determine whether or not violence in media leads directly to youth violence, studies have shown that playing video games increases aggressive thoughts and behaviors. Violent video games not only escalate aggressive behaviors, but they also increase angry thoughts as well as raise the heart rate and blood pressure of participants. Meanwhile, these video games decrease "helping behaviors" and reduce feelings of empathy. Much more, violent video games users tend to interact with other aggressive teens, which makes them feel accepted and validated for their thoughts and feelings. While video games often get the most attention, violence in the media is not limited to video games. Media violence can also include the internet, television, magazines, movies, music, advertising, social media and more. Basically, media consists of anything your teen sees, hears and interacts with.

COMMUNITIES AND NEIGHBORHOODS

Where teens live can also have an impact on them and lead them to act more aggressively. The CDC points to several community risk factors for youths' violence including demolished economic opportunities, high levels of crime and socially disorganized neighborhoods. Additionally, youth violence can become a form of "street justice" in response to lack of police protection in some neighborhood, then these teens attempt to secure the neighborhood by using violence as a way of bringing order to the area. As a result, teens violence often manifests as gang violence, turf wars, gun wars and other types of violence.

When teens live in a socio-economically challenged environment, they may feel like their only option for survival is to join a gang or to engage in violence. When this line of thinking is the norm, teens are likely to act aggressively and participate in violent behaviors.

DOMESTIC VIOLENCE AND CHILD ABUSE

Children who live with violence in the home learn by example and can become violent people as they grow up. They also are likely to experience teen dating violence, either as a victim or as an aggressor. Other contributing factors include harsh parenting styles, doing with chaos in the home, neglect and rejection. Each of these situations can lead to teens' violence because of lack of stability and structure in the home. Being violent gives teens a feeling of power and control, something they lack at home.

To combat this risk, it is important that parents consider their parenting style and make adjustments in order to reduce the likelihood of seeing violence in their teens' lives later. Educators can lend support by offering parenting workshops.

INSUFFICIENT PARENTAL SUPERVISION

When parents do not provide adequate supervision, teens do not have the resources needed to make good choices or to recognize risks. Consequently, these teens tend to make friends with the wrong people, take unnecessary risks and experiment with things an involved parent could not allow. When parents are too permissive, their kids often have no motivation to do well in school and may even stop caring about their future. As a whole, teenagers need fair and firm discipline and consistent interaction and directions, with and from their parents. When parents take an active role in their teens' lives, it reduces the likelihood of teens violence.

Peer Pressure

Peer pressure plays a pivotal role in youth violence, because kids are more likely to engage in risky or violent behaviors when they act as a group. Teens who normally would not be aggressive or violent on their own often feel empowered when in a group. Additionally, teens are more likely to be violent or aggressive when they feel pressured. They also may become violent in order to maintain their place in the group. Peer pressure can lead teens to engage in risk-taking behaviors.

Traumatic Events

Dealing with traumatic events also can cause violent behavior in teens. For instance, teens who lose a friend in a car accident that they also were involved in often get angry at the fact that they were the ones that lived. Because anger is a normal stage of grief, a violent outburst from these teens may seem justified. But while anger is a normal emotion, it is abnormal to be violent towards another person. When violence occurs, it should always be addressed. Teens who exhibit signs of post-traumatic stress disorder (PTSD) may be prone to violence, but if left untreated, can manifest in significantly violent situations.

Mental Illness

Mental illness is another cause of violence among teens. Teens' mental illness sometimes hides behind other causes of youth violence. For instance, a teen with bipolar disorder may be using drugs. If this teen becomes violent, the drug use could hide the fact that the bipolar illness is part of the cause. For this reason, it is important that teens engaging in violent behaviors are evaluated for a mental illness. By treating the entire person, rather than just the symptoms, you are more likely to reduce the risk of additional violent outbursts.

Chapter 7

Mood Expression

Parents should be aware of the signs and symptoms their children express. They should be able to differentiate between expected behaviors and what might be signs of depression or stress. Nigeria parents not all are fond of shouting at their children or beating instead of being closer to the child. There is no test to identify the child problems and seek for help. It is about time for young mothers to learn to cope and most importantly be aware of the children's typical behavior knowing too well that each child is unique and different in nature. Parents should be aware knowing that each abnormal behavior of the teens has its own symptoms. When they start to have excessive sad or low energy. They look confused and have poor concentration as a result with poor school performance. Parents should pay attention and stop calling them names such as "foolish, good for nothing, lazy..."

Mood Change:

When the teen starts to have extreme mood changes that are uncontrollable, and anger as such as avoiding people, parents should pay attention and stop labelling them. Lacking parental support increase their irritability and anger. *The Internalized Stigma Mental Illness Inventory-29(ISMI-29) mentioned a few categories of self-stigma.* The parents who are giving their children 'names' become stigma. These are the barriers for recovery as the result is an increase in depression and a reduce self-esteem and empowerment. Parents should understand the power of self-stigma and lack of understanding may result in a worse outcome. These are the barrier for recovery as result increase depression, reduce self-esteem, and empowerment. Parents should understand the power of self-stigma and lack of understanding may result worse outcome.

Nigeria societies are making it worse with the youth to have job and support themselves, many of them completely depend on family support. There are certain families who are poor and are getting poorer and there are rich families who are richer and are getting richer.

Do Not Care Attitude

Teens' violence is an extreme form of aggression resulting into physical harm, injury, or death. Since violence among teens is gradually taking the lead in our society today, it is necessary to consider the following points as possible solutions. Adults should stop this "do not care" attitude. These children are our future hope. It may affect the generation to come.

Early Intervention:

Early intervention plays an important role in keeping minors from embarking on a life of crime. Parents should offer adequate supervision over their general life, friends, association, and companies kept. They should also offer simple advice to these young ones, paying much attention to their opinions and trying as much as possible to make them feel loved.

Swift Justice For Young Offenders:

Teens who engage in violent act should be dealt with as quickly as possible. This helps to inculcate in them the sense of justice. It is important that juvenile justice is applied to tame teens who feel that there is no way of punishing people who are below age 18. This act will help prevent re-offending by the teens.

Personalized Approach:

Every young person is different and deserves support that is specifically tailored to them. For instance, an aggressive person can be asked to attend a course to learn how to cope with and control aggression. School teachers should know and give recommendations to parents or those adults involving in their lives.

Training And Education Programs:

The organization of training programs aimed at educating and keeping teens busy. It can go a long way to help the situation of teens violence thus, "an idle man is devil's workshop." So, when these teens are occupied with different activities, they tend to work together as a team rather than tearing each other apart on violence.

Tackling Problem Gangs of Teens:

Dealing with problem gangs of teens is one of the things governments should do to alleviate teens' violence. It should investigate specific groups and their individual members. What works best is a combination of care, punitive, education and employment measures. The government should do more than simply setting limits by imposing penalties on teens who have committed a crime. It is also important to offer young people the prospect of work or education. This will keep them from embarking on a life of violence. The integrated approach designed to tackle gangs of youth at local levels should be coordinated by the municipality in collaboration with the police, the public prosecution service and the ministry of security and justice.

CHAPTER 8

Conclusion

Violence is ubiquitous in the Nigerian society. In fact, the most frequently reported stressor in the lives of Nigerian youth is exposure to violence. Depending on one's sex, social class, community and religion, different forms of exposure to violence are more common. For example, from this study, most of the youths have been exposed to violence either in their community, school or in the household.

Exposures to certain types of violence increase the risk of experiencing other forms of violence (Krug, Mercy, Dahlberg, & Zwi, 2002). In communities with high rates of violence, it is likely for an individual to experience violence across multiple settings (Lambert, Nylund-Gibson, Copeland-Linder, & Ialongo, 2010). Yet, much of the research on exposure to violence does not account for unique patterns of exposure, and instead, treats different patterns of exposure similarly (Wright, 1998). In other words, studying everyone's violent experience in isolation may not adequately represent that individual's experience. By identifying youth who report similar types of exposure to violence classes, we may be able to develop better interventions to help youth cope with stressful life events and mitigate the negative repercussions the exposures may cause.

Researchers often state that exposure to violence is a risk factor for later violent perpetration and victimization, but this assertion has not been tested adequately. The 2001 Surgeon General's Report states: *"Studies have shown that adolescents exposed to violence are more likely to engage in violent acts,"* and then goes on to cite several studies, none of which tested this relationship (pg. 1902).

Cited in the report Fagan & Wilkinson (1998), the researchers discuss how exposure to violence should, theoretically, lead to violence given a script framework, but they did not actually conduct such a study (Fagan & Wilkinson, 1998). Another cited study in the report linked exposure to violence to symptoms of psychological trauma, but not too violent behaviors (Singer, Anglin, Song, & Lunghofer, 1995). Other researchers that are frequently cited when linking exposure to violence with subsequent violent behaviors have yielded inconsistent results (Finkelhor et al., 2005) with several researchers reporting no significant relationships (Feigelman, Howard, Li, & Cross, 2000). These inconsistencies may result from studies of varying timeframes and measurement. (Copeland-Linder, Lambert & Lalongo, 2010).

References

1 William Goodwin, Teen Violence 1998 by Lucent Books, Inc, San Diego, CA Printed in the U.S.A. p6

2 Hussey JM, Chang JJ, Kotch JB (2006) Child maltreatment in the United States: prevalence, risk factors, and adolescent health consequences. Pediatrics 118(3):933–942

3 Bair-Merritt MH, Blackstone M, Feudtner C (2006) Physical health outcomes of childhood exposure to intimate partner violence: a systematic review. Pediatrics 117(2):e278–e290

4 Eaton DK et al (2008) Youth risk behavior surveillance—United States, 2007. MMWR Surveill Summ 57(4):1–131

5 Buka SL et al (2001) Youth exposure to violence: prevalence, risks, and consequences. Am J Orthopsychiatry 71(3):298–310

6 Cunradi CB (2009) Intimate partner violence among Hispanic men and women: the role of drinking, neighborhood disorder, and acculturation-related factors. Violence Vict 24(1):83–97

7 Kessler RC, Davis CG, Kendler KS (1997) Childhood adversity and adult psychiatric disorder in the US National Comorbidity Survey. Psychol Med 27(5):1101–1119

McCabe KM et al (2005) The relation between violence exposure and conduct problems among adolescents: a prospective study. Am J Orthopsychiatry 75(4):575–584

8 Covey, H. C., Menard, S., & Franzese, R. J. (2013). Effects of adolescent physical abuse, exposure to neighborhood violence, and witnessing parental violence on adult socioeconomic status. Child Maltreatment, 1077559513477914.

9 Berton, M. W., & Stabb, S. D. (1996). Exposure to violence and post-traumatic stress disorder in urban adolescents. Adolescence, 31(122), 489.

10 Wolfe, D. A., Crooks, C. V., Lee, V., McIntyre-Smith, A., & Jaffe, P. G. (2003). The effects of children's exposure to domestic violence: A meta-analysis and critique. Clinical Child and Family Psychology Review, 6(3), 171–187.

11 Mari JJ, de Mello MF, Figueira I. The impact of urban violence on mental health. Rev Bras de Psiquiatr. 2008;30(3):183-4.

12 Krug EG, Dahlberg LL, Mercy JA, Zwi AB, Lozano R. World report on violence and health. Geneva: World Health Organization; 2002.

13 PAHO. Health situation in the americas: basic indicators. Washington, DC: Pan American Health Organization; 2007.

[14] William Goodwin, Teen Violence 20-21

[15] Ibid 21-22

[16] Holden, G. W. (1998). Introduction: The development of research into another consequence of family violence. In E. W. Holden, R. Geffner, & E. N. Jouriles (Eds.), Children exposed to marital violence: Theory, research, and applied issues (pp. 1–20). Washington, DC: American Psychological Association

[17] Mohr, W. K., Lutz, M. J. N., Fantuzzo, J. W., & Perry, M. A. (2000). Children exposed to family violence: A review of empirical research from a developmental–ecological perspective. Trauma, Violence, and Abuse, 1, 264–283.

[18] Edleson, J. L. (1999). Children's witnessing of adult domestic violence. Journal of Interpersonal Violence, 14, 839–870.

[19] William Goodwin, Teen Violence 22

[20] Bandura, A. (1973). Aggression: A social learning analysis.

[21] Huesmann, L. R. (1988). An information processing model for the development of aggression. Aggressive Behavior, 14(1), 13–24.

[22] Lynch, M., & Cicchetti, D. (1998). An ecological-transactional analysis of children and contexts: The longitudinal interplay among child maltreatment, community violence, and children's symptomatology. Development and Psychopathology, 10(02), 235–257.

[23] Kliewer, W., Lepore, S. J., Oskin, D., & Johnson, P. D. (1998). The role of social and cognitive processes in children's adjustment to community violence. Journal of Consulting and Clinical Psychology, 66(1), 199.

[24] Achenbach, T. M. (1991). Manual for the Child Behavior Checklist/4-18 and 1991 profile.

[25] Angst, J., Gamma, A., Gastpar, M., Lépine, J.-P., Mendlewicz, J., & Tylee, A. (2002). Gender differences in depression. European Archives of Psychiatry and Clinical Neuroscience, 252(5), 201–209.

[26] Margolin, G., & Gordis, E. B. (2000). The effects of family and community violence on children. Annual Review of Psychology, 51(1), 445–479.

[27] Gorman-Smith, D., Henry, D. B., & Tolan, P. H. (2004). Exposure to community violence and violence perpetration: The protective effects of family functioning. Journal of Clinical Child & Adolescent Psychology, 33(3), 439–449.

[28] Cooley-Quille, M., Boyd, R. C., Frantz, E., & Walsh, J. (2001). Emotional and behavioral impact of exposure to community violence in inner-city adolescents. Journal of Clinical Child & Adolescent Psychology, 30(2), 199–206.

Copeland-Linder, N., Lambert, S. F., & Lalongo, N. S. (2010). Community Violence, Protective Factors, and Adolescent Mental Health: A profile analysis. *Journal of Clinical Child & Adolescent Psychology, 39(21) 176-186*

[29] Gaylord-Harden, N. K., Cunningham, J. A., & Zelencik, B. (2011). Effects of exposure to community violence on internalizing symptoms: does desensitization to violence occur in African American youth? Journal of Abnormal Child Psychology, 39(5), 711–719.